PORN ADDITION

FOR WOMEN

Ultimate guide to stop porn addiction fast, (a comprehensive step by step guide to overcome porn addiction in 7 days)

LAUREN D STEPHENS

TABLE OF CONTENTS

Porn addiction for women

INTRODUCTION

It's easy to underestimate the influence of seemingly innocuous habits in a society saturated with digital graphics. For many women, the seductive attraction of online pornographic content may turn into a quiet battle—an addiction with effects that reach far beyond the bounds of a computer. Consider a lady wandering a virtual maze, finding refuge in pixels and transient fancies. She had no idea that this seemingly innocent getaway is actually a covert captor entangling her in a web of dependency.

In this guide, we will go on a quest to unravel the complicated fabric of female porn addiction. Meet Sarah, an alias for many people dealing with this unseen foe. We dig into the complexities of addiction—the quiet battles conducted within the mind and the significant ramifications on personal well-being and relationships—through her narrative and the tales of others. This book is a lifeline, providing insights, techniques, and empowerment to break free from the bonds of addiction and regain a life of true connection and purpose. Let the path to freedom begin.

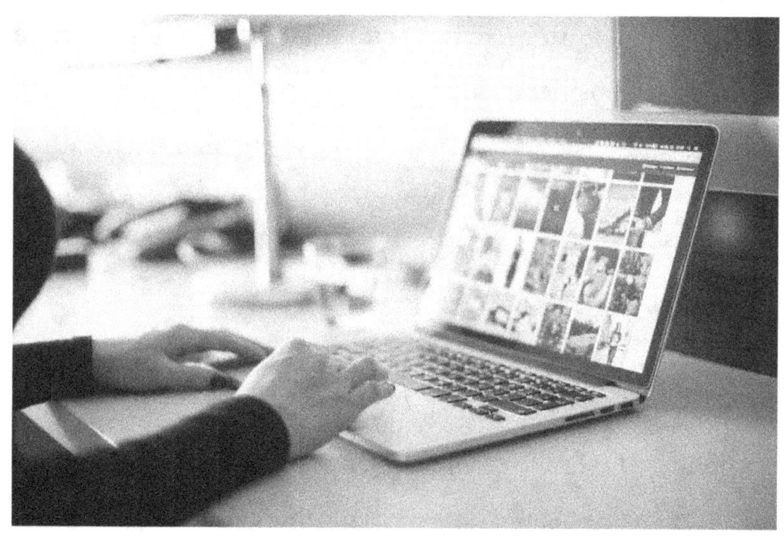

Chapter 1

Understanding Porn Addiction

Porn addiction has infiltrated different demographics in the digital era, when access to sexual content is simply a click away, defying established ideas. While porn addiction has typically been identified with men, the quiet struggle of women ensnared in the web of porn addiction is an often underestimated and stigmatized reality. We hope to shed light on the nuances that underpin the phenomena by exploring the multifaceted environment of female porn addiction.

Defining Porn Addiction:

Before we can understand the complexities of porn addiction in women, we must first define the notion. Porn addiction is an obsessive and harmful practice that interferes with everyday life, not just an enjoyment. This can emerge as an excessive dependency on explicit content in women, leading to a variety of emotional, psychological, and relationship issues.

Prevalence Among Women:

Contrary to popular belief, women make up a sizable proportion of people suffering from porn addiction. Societal expectations frequently disregard or misinterpret this reality, adding to the silence concerning female porn issues. Understanding the prevalence of this problem is critical for dispelling myths and creating a supportive atmosphere for individuals afflicted.

Psychological and Emotional Aspects:

The psychological and emotional underpinnings of female porn addiction are frequently complex. Many women seek sanctuary in the fantasy realm provided by adult content as a coping method. Understanding the multidimensional nature of addiction and establishing successful therapeutic options require unraveling these emotional connections.

Meet Emily: A Narrative Perspective:

Consider Emily, a fictitious figure who represents the silent struggle of innumerable women. Initially benign, her ventures into internet pornographic content evolved into a covert dependency. Emily's narrative is a kaleidoscope of emotions, alternating between escapist and the brutal reality of addiction's effects. We get insight into the internal difficulties and exterior consequences that define the path of a lady ensnared in the web of porn addiction via her experiences.

The Effect on Mental Health:

Understanding the mental health consequences of porn addiction is critical. Women who are going through this battle frequently experience worry, guilt, and a skewed self-image. The guilt associated with such practices can worsen pre-existing mental health issues, producing a vicious cycle that deepens the addiction.

Navigating the Societal Landscape:

Societal norms and expectations shape the experience of female porn addiction significantly. The stigma associated with this illness can lead to seclusion, preventing women from getting treatment or freely expressing their concerns. In order to build empathy and understanding, it is necessary to challenge cultural stereotypes.

Breaking preconceptions:

Breaking preconceptions is critical in breaking down the obstacles that inhibit women from recognizing and addressing their addiction. Women of diverse ages, backgrounds, and relationship statuses may find themselves confronted with this issue. Recognizing the variety of persons impacted is critical for the development of inclusive support networks.

Understanding Porn Addiction in Women:

Understanding porn addiction in women is about helping individuals to retake control over their life. Recognizing the distinct elements that contribute to addiction enables targeted therapies and support networks. It's a voyage of self-discovery, endurance, and, eventually, freedom from the bonds of addiction.

The narrative in this extensive examination of understanding porn addiction in women is one of strength, not victimhood. We open the way for empathy, awareness, and practical ways to help women towards a road of healing and meaningful connection by peeling back the layers of this complicated issue. The following chapters of this guide will go into further detail on spotting warning signals and risks, investigating fundamental causes, and giving effective techniques for control and recovery. The path to emancipation continues.

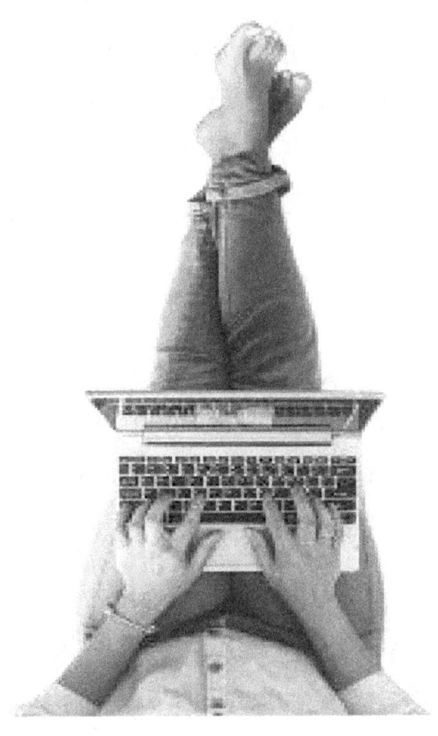

Discuss the prevalence of porn addiction among women.

Porn addiction is frequently regarded via a gendered lens in the addiction landscape, with pervasive misconceptions supporting the perception that it exclusively affects males. A more comprehensive view of this problem, on the other hand, shows a significant and frequently underestimated reality: the persistent incidence of porn addiction among women.

Confronting Stereotypes:

For too long, societal stereotypes and cultural standards have depicted porn addiction as primarily a male problem, obscuring the realities of women dealing with this hidden epidemic. Breaking free from these preconceptions is critical for recognizing the varied population impacted by porn addiction and creating an atmosphere in which women feel safe seeking assistance and support.

The Rise of internet Access:

The internet era has brought unprecedented access to graphic information, redefining conventional gender roles in addiction. Women, like males, find themselves navigating a virtual terrain that provides both anonymity and accessibility. The frequency of porn addiction among women has increased due to the availability of internet pornographic content.

Underreported and stigmatized:

Despite its ubiquity, porn addiction among women is usually unreported, owing to cultural stigmas and the topic's taboo nature. Women may be hesitant to discuss their difficulties for fear of being judged or misunderstood. This unwillingness to discuss the subject publicly maintains the myth that women are less prone to porn addiction, adding to the underestimating of its prevalence.

Affected Demographics are Diverse:

Porn addiction does not discriminate based on age, background, or relationship status. Women from all areas of life, of all ages and ethnic origins, find themselves ensnared in the web of addiction. Recognizing the variety of people impacted is essential for designing tailored treatments and support systems that address the specific needs of various demographic groups.

Relationship Impact:

The prevalence of porn addiction among women has far-reaching consequences for relationships. Recognizing the possible impact on heterosexual and LGBTQ+ relationships as cultural attitudes change is critical. The secrecy around women's porn troubles may strain relationships, weakening trust and communication. Understanding these interactions is critical for providing comprehensive care.

The media's presentation of idealized body images and unrealistic sexual settings can lead to the development of porn addiction in women. Pursuit of unachievable ideals, as maintained by explicit material, may function as a coping mechanism for underlying anxieties, impacting the incidence of addiction.

The Importance of studies and knowledge:

The underrepresentation of women in porn addiction studies exacerbates the lack of public knowledge about its prevalence. Advancing research programs that especially investigate women's experiences can help to a more thorough knowledge of the issue, dispelling myths and encouraging empathy.

Explore the psychological and emotional aspects of addiction.

To really understand and handle the complexities of female porn addiction, we must venture into the unknown territory of the psychological and emotional factors that drive this complicated issue.

For many women, porn addiction begins as a type of escapism, a retreat into a universe of fantasy that momentarily protects them from the hardships of reality. Recognizing the function of explicit content as a coping technique is necessary for understanding the psychological origins. Women who are under stress, worry, or emotional anguish may find relief in the illusory world portrayed by adult literature.

Impact on Self-Perception:

Porn addiction has a psychological impact on self-perception. Exposure to idealized bodies and unrealistic settings can affect a woman's sense of self, resulting to anxieties and a poor body image. As the addiction worsens, the gap between the idealized personas in explicit content and one's own self-image grows wider, continuing a cycle of guilt and further entrenching the addiction.

Exploring the emotional implications of porn addiction necessitates diving into the underlying mechanisms that drive this behavior. Unresolved emotional difficulties, prior traumas, or unmet emotional needs may all lead to the use of explicit content for self-soothing or diversion. Recognizing and managing these emotional triggers is critical for building successful intervention and rehabilitation techniques.

Dynamics of Shame and Guilt:

The emotional landscape of porn addiction is frequently marred by chronic emotions of shame and guilt. As women struggle with the stigma attached to this type of addiction, these feelings become powerful hurdles to obtaining assistance. Understanding the interaction between shame and guilt is critical for building a supportive atmosphere that promotes openness and aids in the healing process.

Relationship Impact:

The emotional implications of porn addiction affect interpersonal relationships in addition to individual issues.

Addiction's secrecy and guilt may strain relationships, weakening trust and intimacy. Exploring the emotional dynamics of romantic and family relationships is critical for designing techniques that address not just individual healing but also the repair of relational ties.

Cognitive Distortions and harmful habits:

Addiction is frequently characterized psychologically by cognitive distortions and harmful behavioral habits. Women may have skewed attitudes about intimacy, relationships, and their own value, which can perpetuate the addiction cycle. Recognizing and confronting these cognitive distortions is an important step toward altering thought habits and cultivating a healthier mentality.

To summarize, in order to successfully address and help women in overcoming porn addiction, it is critical to investigate the psychological and emotional factors that contribute to and perpetuate this complicated problem. Recognizing the function of escapism, comprehending its influence on self-perception, and investigating underlying emotional reasons are critical components of a comprehensive therapeutic strategy. We prepare the way for a journey of self-discovery and healing by peeling back the layers of shame, guilt, and cognitive distortions—one that goes beyond breaking free from addiction to recovering a positive and powerful sense of self.

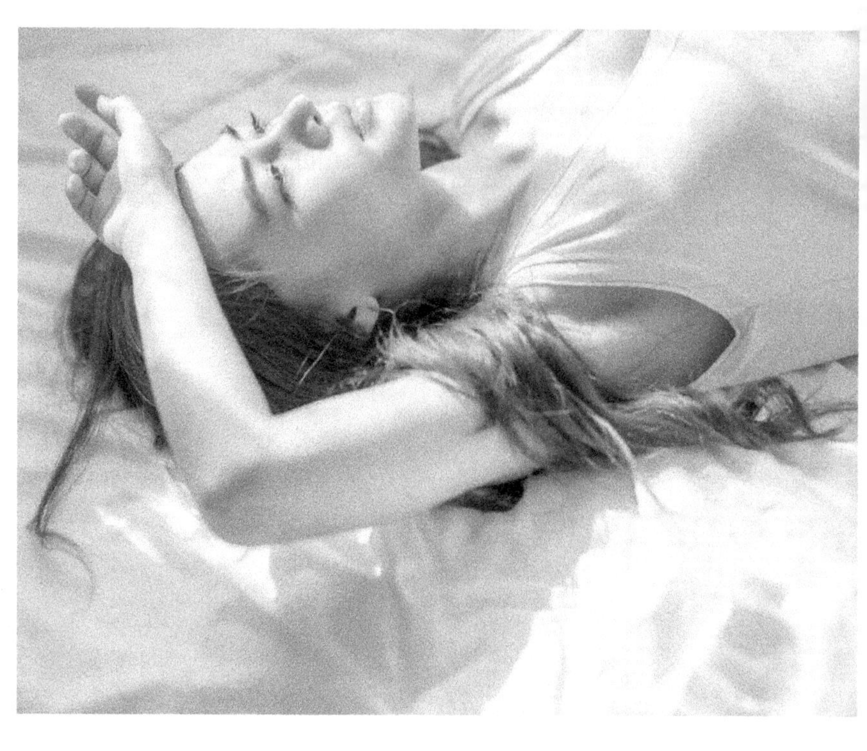

Chapter 2

Recognizing the Signs and Dangers

Porn addiction throws a subtle shadow in the quiet hallways of women's difficulties, frequently avoiding detection. The second chapter attempts to expose these shadows by giving a guide to recognizing the indications and hazards of porn addiction in women, creating awareness that is critical for prompt intervention.

Subtle Behavioral Changes:

Recognizing porn addiction in women necessitates a detailed comprehension of subtle behavioral changes. As the addiction takes hold, a formerly robust social life may fade, leading to greater isolation. Changes in sleep habits, mood fluctuations, and a progressive withdrawal from formerly cherished hobbies may indicate a deeper struggle. Paying attention to these minor adjustments is the first step toward detecting the addiction's insidious nature.

Secrecy and concealment:

Women who are addicted to porn frequently become skilled at disguising their behaviors, building webs of secrecy around their acts. Frequent deleting of browser history, usage of private browsing modes, or increased protectiveness of electronic equipment might all be signs of a wish to conceal the addiction. Recognizing these privacy safeguards is critical in revealing the covert character of the conflict.

Relationship Impact:

One of the poignant symptoms is in the arena of relationships. Porn addiction may sever intimate and trusting friendships. Women may retreat emotionally and struggle to connect closely with partners. Recognizing these relational pressures, such as a reduction in communication or increased tension, is critical for comprehending the addiction's interpersonal consequences.

intake Escalation:

As addiction tightens its grasp, there is frequently a visible increase in the intake of explicit content. What previously pleased no longer does, leading to an increasing need for more severe content. Recognizing this process is critical for comprehending the changing nature of the addiction and the importance of prompt intervention to prevent future escalation.

Impact on Mental Health:

Porn addiction has a significant impact on mental health. Signs of discomfort might include increased anxiety, sadness, or a general reduction in well-being. Recognizing these mental health markers is critical because they provide insights into the psychological problems that women confront while navigating the maze of addiction.

Neglect of obligations:

Neglect of obligations is a common warning sign. Women who are addicted to porn may have their everyday lives disturbed when commitments at work, in the family, or in personal hobbies take a second place. Recognizing the abandonment of once-cherished obligations reveals the extent to which the addiction has permeated all facets of life.

Denial and Resistance to Intervention:

The individual's refusal to acknowledge the situation is an often-overlooked symptom. When faced with the addiction, denial, defensiveness, or avoidance might suggest a serious issue with acceptance. Recognizing these protective strategies is critical for handling the issue with care and compassion, establishing an environment in which women feel supported rather than criticized.

Physical and Emotional implications:

Porn addiction has physical and emotional implications that transcend beyond the digital sphere. Recognizing indications like physical discomfort, weariness, or a significant reduction in emotional well-being offers a comprehensive picture of the toll this addiction has on the individual.

Identify common signs of porn addiction in women.

Recognizing common indications is critical in the maze of women's experiences with porn addiction. The second chapter attempts to peel back the layers of secrecy, giving a detailed guide to identifying the minor clues that may indicate the presence of this covert conflict.

Modified Social Behavior:

Changes in social conduct are sometimes one of the first indicators. Women who are addicted to porn may withdraw from social activities or isolate themselves from friends and relatives. Reduced interest in previously enjoyed social contacts may be an early sign of the addiction's growing influence.

Increased Secrecy and Privacy Protection:

Women who are addicted to porn become skilled at disguising their behaviors. An increase in covert conduct, such as constantly cleaning browsing history, using private browsing modes, or aggressively guarding electronic gadgets, is a strong indication of a wish to conceal the addiction. Recognizing these privacy safeguards is critical to comprehending the clandestine character of the conflict.

Increase in Consumption:

An increase in the intake of explicit content is a telltale symptom of addiction growth. What formerly pleased women may no longer do so, prompting them to seek out more extreme content. Recognizing this shift in consumption habits gives insights on the changing nature of the addiction as well as the need of intervention.

Sleep Pattern Alterations:

The allure of pornographic content might interfere with natural sleep habits. Women suffering from porn addiction may find themselves up late at night, immersed in internet material. The regret and humiliation associated with addiction, on the other hand, might lead to sleeplessness. Recognizing sleep disruptions is critical for understanding the influence on overall well-being.

Intimate Relationship Tensions:

Porn addiction has repercussions in close relationships. A reduction in emotional closeness, problems connecting with a spouse, or an overall tension in the relationship may be signs. Recognizing these relationship alterations is critical for comprehending the addiction's interpersonal repercussions.

Escapist Conduct:

Addiction is frequently used as a type of getaway from life's difficulties. Women may seek out graphic information to relieve tension, worry, or emotional anguish. Recognizing an escapist tendency is crucial for understanding the underlying emotional factors that contribute to the dependency on porn.

Failure to Meet Responsibilities:

As porn addiction grips women, they may disregard their obligations at work, at home, or in personal hobbies. Recognizing a reduction in the accomplishment of once-cherished commitments reveals the extent to which the addiction has permeated numerous facets of life.

Emotional Distress and Mood Swings:

Porn addiction has an emotional toll in the form of mood swings and increased mental anguish. Women who consume explicit information may have significant feelings of guilt, humiliation, or worry. awareness the psychological challenges connected with addiction requires an awareness of these emotional changes.

Opposition to Intervention:

The individual's refusal to acknowledge the problem is an often-overlooked symptom. When faced with the addiction, denial, defensiveness, or avoidance might suggest a serious issue with acceptance. Recognizing these protective strategies is critical for handling the issue with care and compassion, establishing an environment in which women feel supported rather than criticized.

Discuss the negative effects of porn addiction on mental health, relationships, and overall well-being.

The ramifications of women's experiences with porn addiction weave through the fabric of their life, leaving marks on their mental health, relationships, and general well-being. This subchapter digs into the significant and often subtle negative repercussions of addiction, putting light on the complicated tapestry of consequences that accompany the shady journey of addiction.

Influence on Mental Health:

Porn addiction's insidious nature throws a shadow on mental health, impacting women on emotional and psychological levels. Guilt, guilt, and anxiety become unwanted companions, exacerbating the psychological tensions caused by hidden intake of graphic information. Pornographically warped impressions of intimacy lead to a poor self-image, magnifying feelings of inadequacy and prolonging a cycle of emotional discomfort.

As the addiction worsens, a persistent sensation of solitude may develop, leading to increased anxiety and sadness. A chaotic emotional environment is created by the ongoing conflict between the urge for connection and the shame connected with the addiction. Recognizing the emotional toll of the battle is critical for devising therapies that address the emotional complexities of the conflict.

Relationship Effects:

Porn addiction's tentacles reach beyond the person, entwining with the delicate threads of close connections. Addiction concealment may strain communication, damage trust, and disturb emotional connection between couples. The relationship fabric may unravel as women cope with the shame associated with their intake of explicit information, leading to increasing tensions and disputes.

Addiction destroys intimacy, both emotional and physical. Pornographic depictions of unrealistic events can create a schism between lovers, distorting expectations and impeding genuine bonding. Recognizing these relational tensions is critical for comprehending the far-reaching effects of porn addiction on the intricate dynamics of love relationships.

Influence on Overall Well-Being:

Porn addiction has far-reaching consequences for one's general well-being. Women may find themselves ignoring once-cherished obligations when the addiction infiltrates numerous facets of their lives. Work, familial responsibilities, and personal ambitions may suffer as a result of the constant search of explicit content, resulting in a decrease in overall life satisfaction.

Physical health is not immune to the effects of addiction. Sleep disruptions, whether caused by late-night consumption or worry linked with guilt, add to exhaustion and a general sensation of malaise. Neglecting physical health, as well as emotional well-being, results in a comprehensive reduction in total well-being.

Recognizing the harmful repercussions of porn addiction is the first step toward creating empathy and understanding. This subchapter attempts to provide readers with a thorough understanding of the multiple effects of addiction by unwinding the threads of mental health issues, relationship pressures, and a reduction in general well-being. We prepare the path for therapies that address not only the behavior but also the delicate tapestry of emotions and connections entwined within as we negotiate the complexity of this battle.

Highlight the importance of early recognition and intervention.

The importance of early detection and quick intervention in the complicated dance of porn addiction cannot be emphasized. Chapter 2.2 dives into the importance of recognizing warning signals and acting early, bringing light on how these critical acts may change the trajectory of an individual's struggle and pave the way for a road of healing and recovery.

Mitigating Escalation:

One of the most important reasons for early detection is to avoid escalation. Porn addiction, like many other behavioral illnesses, progresses over time. What appears to be a little conflict may quickly escalate into a widespread and all-encompassing force. Early detection allows for therapies while addictive behaviors are still developing, reducing the danger of the behavior becoming profoundly established.

Individuals and their support networks can apply methods to stop the progression of addiction by recognizing the indicators before it reaches advanced stages. Timely interventions can break the addictive cycle, avoiding further entrenchment and paving the way for a more manageable route to recovery.

Protecting Mental Health:

Early detection is critical in protecting mental health. Porn addiction has a severe influence on mental health that worsens as the addiction grows. Guilt, shame, and anxiety can become exhausting, resulting to increased stress and the possible development of underlying mental health disorders.

By detecting the warning symptoms early, the psychological toll may be addressed before it becomes entrenched. This not only helps the individual navigate the emotional difficulties of addiction, but it also helps to avoid the development of more serious mental health issues. Early treatments, such as counseling and therapeutic support, can help people cope with emotional discomfort and build resilience.

Preserving Relationship Resilience:

Intervening early in the course of porn addiction is critical for preserving relationship resilience. Strains and fractures may arise as the addiction infiltrates the dynamics of close relationships. Early identification allows for open discussion between partners, creating a climate in which the impact of the addiction on the relationship may be handled sensitively and understandingly.

Couples should emphasize marital well-being by noticing indications such as changes in intimacy, communication habits, and emotional distance. Relationship counseling or therapy customized to the specific issues provided by porn addiction can be undertaken, providing a proactive approach to sustaining relationship bonds.

Preventing loneliness and Stigma:

Early detection helps to avoid the severe loneliness and stigma that can accompany porn addiction. Recognizing the warning flags early provides for a more open and compassionate approach within support networks. Individuals in the early stages of addiction are more inclined to reveal their troubles when they are treated with compassion rather than condemnation.

Isolation prevention is critical because it provides a sense of connection and lowers the guilt associated with addiction. Early on, support from friends, family, or mental health experts may be mobilized, forming a network that mitigates the isolating effects of addiction and encourages the individual to seek assistance without fear of stigma.

Making Treatment Pathways Easier:

Early detection makes treatment paths easier and more manageable. Addiction therapies, whether in the form of counseling, support groups, or therapeutic modalities, are frequently more successful when started early. Individuals may be more open to therapies when behavioral patterns are still emerging, making the process of behavior change and recovery more reachable.

Furthermore, early detection allows for a less complicated therapy landscape. The longer an addiction endures, the more it becomes entwined with numerous elements of life, needing more thorough and lengthy therapies. Recognition in a timely manner allows for focused treatments, perhaps expediting the treatment process and increasing the probability of effective recovery.

Encourage Personal Empowerment:

Early awareness allows individuals to take charge of their rehabilitation process. Individuals are positioned as active participants in their own healing process by recognizing the signals and intervening early. This acknowledgement provides a feeling of agency, motivating individuals to seek assistance, engage in self-reflection, and handle the issues provided by porn addiction constructively.

Encouragement of personal empowerment via early acknowledgment is critical in developing a resilient and self-efficacy mentality. It supports the idea that recovery is possible and that with the correct support and treatments, people can negotiate the intricacies of addiction.

Finally, the significance of early detection and intervention in porn addiction cannot be emphasized. Early detection becomes a cornerstone in the process toward recovery by limiting escalation, conserving mental health, maintaining interpersonal resilience, reducing isolation and stigma, promoting simpler treatment paths, and fostering personal empowerment.

This chapter acts as a guidepost, encouraging readers to take a proactive position by detecting the indicators of addiction and acting in the early stages, exposing a route toward recovery, resilience, and empowerment.

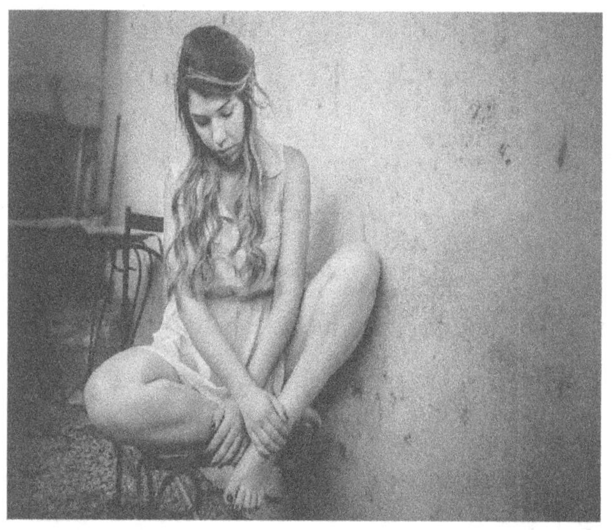

Exploring the Root Causes

As we proceed further into the intricate topography of women's issues with porn addiction, Chapter 3 delves into the underlying reasons of this complex phenomena. Understanding the causes of addiction is critical for establishing specialized therapies and support systems that address the particular circumstances that contribute to a dependency on explicit material.

Cultural Influences:

The cultural context has a profound impact on the landscape of porn addiction among women. The normalization of explicit content consumption is aided by societal expectations, conventions, and media portrayals of sexuality. Cultural taboos surrounding frank sexuality talks may lead women to seek consolation in the anonymity of online adult material, establishing a dependency that can lead to addiction.

Investigating sociocultural impacts entails deciphering the intricate interaction of cultural expectations, gender norms, and messages about female sexuality. Understanding the cultural roots that may lead to porn addiction allows therapies to be designed to confront and alter these effects, producing a healthy sexual connection.

Personal Experiences and Trauma:

Personal experiences and trauma frequently affect individual paths. Porn addiction may have origins in prior traumas, unresolved emotions, or unfulfilled emotional needs for certain women. Exploring these personal narratives entails engaging in self-discovery and reflection.

Trauma, whether from childhood or more recent circumstances, can serve as a catalyst for seeking solace and escape in the fantasy world of pornography. Addressing the fundamental reasons entails establishing a safe environment for people to examine and process their unique experiences, which promotes healing and resilience.

Psychological Aspects and Coping skills: The psychological aspects of porn addiction are complex, frequently requiring the development of coping skills to handle life's problems.

Understanding the psychological components necessitates investigating how addiction may be used to escape or cope with stress, worry, or emotional distress.

Women may seek brief relief from life's challenges by turning to explicit content as a method of self-soothing. Untangling these psychological strands allows therapies to be personalized to give alternate coping mechanisms, helping women to address underlying difficulties in healthier ways.

Sexual Expression and Empowerment:

Because sexuality is such an important part of the human experience, it plays a role in the development of porn addiction. Consumption of explicit content may be connected to the exploration of one's own sexuality for certain women. However, cultural stigmas and taboos surrounding female sexual expression may propel this investigation into the shadowy world of addiction.

Exploring the origins of porn addiction in the context of sexual expression entails creating a safe space for women to accept and negotiate their sexuality without shame or condemnation. Empowering women to express their sexuality in ways that are consistent with their beliefs and limits is critical to changing the narrative surrounding sexual empowerment.

Peer and Relationship Influences:

Relationship dynamics and peer influences both contribute to the origins of porn addiction. Women may be attracted into the realm of explicit content as a result of partner preferences, social influences, or a desire to comply to perceived norms within partnerships.

Understanding these factors entails investigating the dynamics of peer interactions as well as the impact of intimate relationships on the development and maintenance of addiction. Interventions may then be created to address relationship issues while encouraging open communication and mutual understanding within relationships.

Investigate potential underlying factors contributing to porn addiction in women.

Chapter 3.2 continues to analyze the probable underlying reasons that weave into the complicated fabric of addiction in the intricate tapestry of women's battles with porn addiction. Understanding these aspects is critical for developing nuanced therapies that address the specific and different foundations of the dependence on explicit material.

Social and Cultural Influences:

Societal and cultural norms have a significant impact on the landscape of porn addiction among women. Investigating these factors entails looking at societal expectations regarding female sexuality, the normalization of explicit content, and the impact of cultural taboos on open sex talks.

Cultural pressures may lead women to seek comfort and discovery in the dark corners of pornography, establishing a dependency that can lead to addiction. Examining these effects allows treatments to be customized to challenge cultural conventions, promote better attitudes regarding female sexuality, and develop a more open discourse.

Individual Experiences and Trauma:

The inquiry into potential underlying variables must cross the very intimate terrain of individual experiences and trauma. Past traumas, whether from childhood or more current occurrences, might become underlying elements motivating women to embrace sexual content as an escapism.

Exploring these unique histories entails providing a safe environment for people to process and recover from emotional scars. Interventions can be tailored to meet the individual requirements resulting from personal trauma, developing resilience and providing alternate outlets for emotional expression and healing.

Psychological Coping strategies:

One of the psychological aspects of porn addiction is the development of coping strategies to deal with life's obstacles. Understanding how addiction acts as a sort of escape or self-soothing in the face of stress, anxiety, or emotional turmoil is required for research into these coping methods.

Women may take refuge in the momentary respite provided by explicit material as a coping method. Interventions can look at different coping techniques, giving women better tools for overcoming psychological problems and resolving underlying concerns.

Societal Stigmas and Sexual Expression:

The research into underlying variables includes societal stigmas as well as the complex dynamics of sexual expression. Female sexuality taboos and societal restrictions may encourage women to pursue their sexual impulses in hidden worlds, contributing to the development of addiction.

It is critical to create an environment in which sexual expression is accepted without shame or criticism. Interventions might try to modify cultural narratives by encouraging women to express their sexuality in ways that are consistent with their beliefs and limits, therefore addressing the fundamental causes of addiction.

Peer Influences and Relationship Dynamics:

The inquiry must traverse the delicate dynamics of relationships and peer influences. Women may be attracted into the realm of explicit content as a result of partner preferences, social influences, or a desire to comply to perceived norms within partnerships.

Exploring communication patterns, power inequalities, and social expectations within intimate partnerships is necessary for understanding the impact of peer and interpersonal influences. Interventions can then be directed at relationship dynamics, encouraging open communication, mutual understanding, and the development of healthy relationships.

Encourage self-reflection and awareness.

As we explore the perilous terrain of porn addiction recovery, Chapter 3.3 encourages women on a journey of self-reflection and awareness. This chapter delves into personal experiences in order to inspire people to look into the mirrors of their souls, unraveling the layers that lead to addiction and cultivating a profound sense of self-awareness.

The transforming Power of Self-Reflection:

Self-reflection is a transforming tool in the recovery path, providing individuals with a safe environment to explore their ideas, feelings, and behaviors with honesty and openness. In order to encourage women to engage on a path of self-reflection, the tools and advice needed to manage the difficult process of introspection must be provided.

Women might begin to disentangle the complicated web of circumstances that contribute to their dependency on explicit content by looking inside. This introspective approach serves as a mirror, reflecting the complexities of personal experiences, cultural influences, and emotional landscapes that define their connection with pornography.

Drawing on Personal Experiences:

When the story of self-reflection is intertwined with personal experiences, it gains depth and resonance. Sharing tales of perseverance, suffering, and epiphanies weaves a web of connection, allowing women to see themselves reflected in the lives of others. Personal accounts offer a road map for navigating the ups and downs of recovery, as well as inspiration and empathy.

Incorporating personal stories entails showcasing the many journeys of women who have faced the difficulties of porn addiction. These anecdotes act as lighthouses, illuminating the path toward self-awareness and healing by sharing victories, challenges, and moments of self-discovery.

Navigating cultural Expectations:

Self-reflection extends beyond personal experiences to include an examination of cultural norms and expectations. Women are urged to think critically about how cultural taboos, societal expectations, and gender roles impact their connection with explicit information. This introspective trip assists individuals in identifying external causes that may have quietly influenced their behaviors and viewpoints.

Personal experiences in the context of society serve as mirrors, reflecting the influence of cultural norms on personal decisions. Women might obtain insight into how social factors may have had a part in the development of their addiction by navigating these thoughts, building a greater knowledge of external pressures.

Uncovering Emotional Wounds:

In the darkness of emotional wounds, self-reflection is a strong lantern. To encourage women to confront previous traumas and unmet emotional needs, a secure and supportive atmosphere must be created. Personal experiences serve as mirrors, reflecting the suffering, resilience, and progress that result from dealing with emotional traumas.

Women can understand the origins of their addiction and begin the recovery process by navigating these emotional landscapes. Personal stories shared in this environment become powerful mirrors, reflecting the transforming potential of admitting and healing emotional scars.

Exploring Coping Mechanisms:

Self-reflection dives into the psychological components of addiction, including coping mechanism exploration. Women are encouraged to consider the function of explicit material as a stress, anxiety, or emotional turmoil coping method. Personal experiences serve as mirrors, revealing how coping techniques may act as both shields and chains.

Women can uncover better coping mechanisms that match with their beliefs and help to overall well-being by navigating these reflections. Personal accounts in this inquiry act as empowerment mirrors, demonstrating the ability to create resilient and adaptable coping techniques.

Fostering Empowerment via insight:

The profound insight that nurtures empowerment is the result of self-reflection and personal experiences. Women are urged to embrace self-reflective disclosures, acknowledging the interconnectivity of personal experiences, cultural influences, emotional scars, and coping methods.

Awareness becomes a mirror, reflecting the courage to face problems and make deliberate decisions. Within this concept, personal narratives function as mirrors of empowerment, reflecting the transforming path from self-reflection to self-awareness.

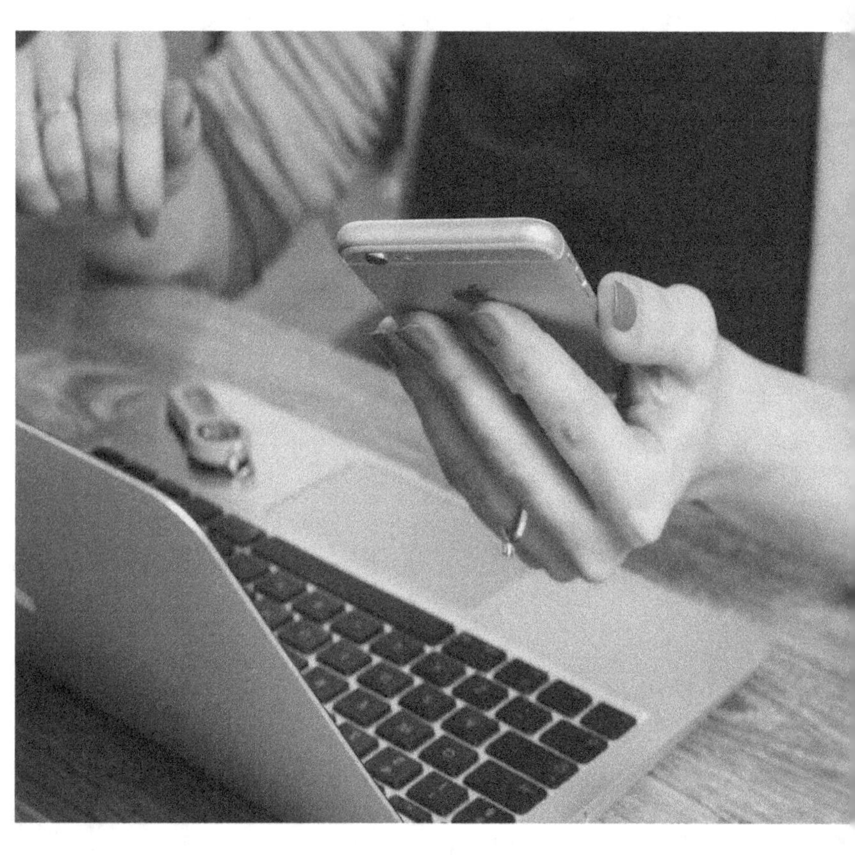

Chapter 4

Strategies for Control

Regaining control in the arena of porn addiction is a difficult road, but it is also one lined with methods that allow women to direct their own path toward recovery. Chapter 4 acts as a guide, revealing a range of options for regaining control and forging a path toward healing, resilience, and self-empowerment.

Cultivating Mindfulness:

Mindfulness is a key method for restoring control. Encouragement of mindfulness in women entails fostering an awareness of the present moment without judgment. Individuals may gain a better knowledge of their thoughts, feelings, and behaviors by practicing mindfulness, laying the groundwork for conscious and empowered decision-making.

Mindfulness serves as a compass, leading women through the treacherous waters of addiction. Meditation, deep breathing exercises, and attentive awareness of triggers all help to the development of this useful method.

Creating Healthy limits:

Regaining control necessitates the creation of healthy limits. Women are encouraged to consider their beliefs, desires, and boundaries, and to express these in their relationships and daily life. Setting defined limits acts as a barrier against the development of addictive habits.

This method entails communicating limits assertively to partners, friends, and oneself. Creating a system of restrictions promotes a sense of control and autonomy, producing an atmosphere conducive to healing.

Creating a Support Network:

The importance of having a support network cannot be emphasized. Connecting with friends, family, and support groups gives a foundation of encouragement and understanding. This network serves as a lifeline, providing support, empathy, and accountability on the road to recovery.

Women are encouraged to share their stories, to rely on their support network during difficult times, and to enjoy their achievements together. Collective awareness provides a potent technique for negotiating the intricacies of addiction.

Seeking Professional counsel:

Seeking professional counsel is a strategic anchor in the drive for control. Therapists, counselors, and addiction experts provide knowledge and tools to the rehabilitation process. Professional advice entails a specialized strategy that addresses the particular features of each woman's addiction battle.

Cognitive-behavioral therapy (CBT) and dialectical behavior therapy (DBT) are therapeutic therapies that provide skills for regulating triggers, confronting erroneous thinking, and establishing healthy coping mechanisms. This cooperation serves as a compass, helping women to long-term rehabilitation.

Using Technology Safeguards:

In today's digital world, technology can be both a blessing and a curse. Using technological protections to reclaim control is a proactive technique for restoring control. Women are urged to use filters, parental controls, or accountability applications to prevent access to sexual content.

This technique entails using technology as an aid in the healing process. Women may retake control of their online experiences by using solutions that encourage responsibility and limit access to triggering content.

Engaging in Healthy Activities:

Engaging in healthy activities is necessary to fill the hole created by addicted behaviors. Control strategies include recognizing and adopting things that provide you joy, contentment, and a sense of success. This might involve pursuing hobbies, engaging in physical activity, or attending community activities.

Healthy activities serve as an anchor, diverting attention away from addictive behaviors and toward experiences that promote general well-being. This method entails establishing a good and nourishing atmosphere that aids in the rehabilitation process.

Accepting Self-Care:

Self-care is a non-negotiable technique on the road to recovery and control. Women are taught to put their physical, emotional, and mental health first. This includes developing habits that nurture the body and mind, such as getting enough sleep, eating well, and exercising regularly.

Self-care becomes a refuge, providing relief from the struggles of rehabilitation. This technique entails accepting the notion that investing in one's own well-being is a strong kind of self-empowerment.

Provide practical tips and strategies for women to gain control over their consumption of porn.

Reclaiming control over your porn intake is a journey that involves both introspection and practical measures. Here are 13 effective and tried-and-true recommendations and tactics for women traversing this route, aimed at enabling individuals to acquire control over their relationship with explicit content.

Self-Reflection as a Basis:

Begin with introspection. Learn about the motives and triggers that lead to porn usage. This introspective journey lays the groundwork for designing focused solutions that are in line with personal goals and beliefs.

Establish Specific Intentions and objectives:

Establish specific intentions and objectives for decreasing or eliminating porn usage. Setting concrete, quantifiable, and realistic goals serves as a road map for success and helps keep the focus on the ultimate aim of achieving control.

Establish and Communicate Boundaries:

Set and communicate clear boundaries for the intake of explicit content. Setting limitations on the time, frequency, and sorts of content accessible is part of this. It is critical to communicate these boundaries clearly to oneself and, if relevant, to partners.

Create a Support Network:

Surround yourself with a network of supporting friends, family, or a support group. Share your objectives with people you can depend on for support, understanding, and accountability. A supportive network gives support during difficult times.

Use Technology Safeguards:

Use technology as an ally. To limit access to explicit content, use filters, parental controls, or accountability applications. These precautions serve as practical obstacles, minimizing the possibility of impulsive consuming.

Engage in Healthy Alternatives:

Look for and participate in activities that provide you joy, fulfillment, and a feeling of success. Whether it's via hobbies, physical activity, or artistic efforts, diverting energy into good alternatives helps to divert attention away from porn viewing.

Mindfulness Techniques:

Incorporate mindfulness activities into your daily life. Meditation, deep breathing, or attentive observation of thoughts and emotions create heightened awareness of triggers and give tools for impulse management.

Create a schedule:

Establish a regular daily schedule that reduces idle time. A well-planned schedule lowers possibilities for impulsive behavior and creates a sense of control over how time is spent, which aids in breaking the habitual consuming cycle.

Educate Yourself:

Arm yourself with information on the impacts of porn usage on mental health and relationships. Understanding the ramifications is a tremendous motivation for change and underlines the urgency of regaining control.

Seek Professional Help:

Seek professional help from therapists, counselors, or addiction experts. Professional counseling provides specific tactics and coping mechanisms adapted to individual requirements, as well as helpful insights for overcoming obstacles.

Recognize and enjoy tiny successes:

Recognize and enjoy tiny successes along the road. Every step toward mastery is a huge accomplishment. Recognizing progress builds confidence and strengthens dedication to the recovery path.

Self-Compassion:

Throughout the process, cultivate self-compassion. Recognize that setbacks are a normal part of any transformation path. Approach obstacles with compassion and understanding, cultivating a pleasant and caring connection with oneself.

Maintain Persistence and Patience:

Gaining control is a long process that needs perseverance and patience. Recognize that significant change takes time and that failures do not define the path. Maintain your focus on the big picture and appreciate your perseverance in the face of adversity.

Finally, these 13 practical recommendations and methods provide a holistic strategy for women looking to take control over their porn usage. These tactics enable individuals to manage the intricacies of addiction with resilience, intentionality, and a revitalized sense of control over their life by combining self-reflection, explicit goal-setting, technology safeguards, mindfulness practices, and professional supervision.

Coping mechanisms for dealing with triggers and urges.

Overcoming porn addiction entails addressing triggers and cravings, significant obstacles that need a robust and planned approach. Here, we look at effective coping methods that can help women deal with these triggers and desires, paving the way for recovery.

Develop Mindfulness Techniques:

Mindfulness is an effective tool for dealing with triggers and impulses. Individuals can notice thoughts and emotions without judgment by growing present-moment awareness. Meditation and mindful breathing are two mindfulness activities that might help you stay grounded and break the reflexive response to stimuli.

Set up a Trigger Journal:

Keeping a trigger notebook can be an effective coping tool. Keep track of triggers, including the feelings, events, and ideas that go with them. This exercise not only increases self-awareness but also gives insights into patterns, allowing people to build focused techniques for dealing with certain triggers.

Implement a Strategy of Pause and Reflection:

When confronted with a trigger or impulse, utilize a pause-and-reflect method. Instead of giving in to the urge, take a conscious pause. Consider your emotions, ideas, and events in relation to the trigger. This moment of thinking interrupts the natural response, allowing you to pick a more deliberate path of action.

Participate in Physical Activity:

Physical activity is an effective way to deal with impulses. Include regular exercise in your regimen since it not only improves your general well-being but also produces endorphins, which work as natural mood boosters. When confronted with a desire, channel the energy into a physical activity to interrupt the cycle.

Create Emergency Distractions:

Prepare a list of emergency diversions for times when you have strong impulses. Engaging activities that attract attention and alter focus are examples of diversions.

Whether it's listening to music, doing a hobby, or going for a stroll, having a repertory of diversions is a useful tool for dealing with difficult situations.

Make Use of Visualization Techniques:

Visualization methods can assist in refocusing thoughts and redirecting concentration. When a trigger occurs, imagine a relaxing, happy situation. Imagine a peaceful natural location, engage in a gratifying activity, or see personal accomplishments. Visualization acts as a mental getaway, helping people to traverse triggers more easily.

Experiment with Progressive Muscle Relaxation:

Progressive muscle relaxation is a method that includes tensing and relaxing distinct muscle groups in a systematic manner. This technique encourages physical and emotional relaxation, assisting individuals in managing stress and anxiety, both of which can lead to cravings. Incorporating progressive muscle relaxation into a daily habit on a regular basis might be a proactive coping tool.

Create a Support System:

Building a solid support network is essential for dealing with triggers and impulses. Share your struggles and solutions with trustworthy friends, family, or a support group. Having people who understand and encourage you provides a safety net during difficult times, offering comfort and drive to keep on track.

Make a list of positive affirmations:

Positive affirmations are an effective strategy for changing cognitive habits. Make a list of affirmations that will help you stay committed to your recovery. When confronted with triggers, repeat these affirmations to fight negative thoughts and fortify your determination. Affirmations promote a positive mental conversation that increases resilience.

Use Therapeutic Techniques:

Therapeutic procedures for dealing with triggers include cognitive-behavioral therapy (CBT), dialectical behavior therapy (DBT), and acceptance and commitment therapy (ACT). These therapy approaches provide practical skills and coping methods that address the underlying beliefs and feelings that contribute to cravings.

Establish and Celebrate Milestones:

Setting goals and appreciating accomplishments is a motivating coping method. Break down the healing process into achievable segments and celebrate your success along the way. During difficult times, milestones act as reminders of resilience and give good reinforcement.

Accept Self-Compassion:

In the face of triggers and cravings, cultivate self-compassion as a guiding principle. Recognize that setbacks are a normal part of the rehabilitation process, and treat yourself with compassion and understanding. Self-compassion cultivates a loving relationship with oneself, laying the groundwork for negotiating the intricacies of addiction.

Prepare for Difficult Situations:

Anticipate difficult circumstances and plan for them ahead of time. This entails recognizing possible triggers and devising particular tactics to deal with these situations. A well-thought-out strategy provides individuals with the skills they need to face obstacles with perseverance and resolve.

Finally, these coping methods offer a full toolset for women looking to handle triggers and impulses while recovering from porn addiction. Individuals can navigate difficult situations by incorporating mindfulness practices, creating a trigger journal, implementing pause-and-reflect strategies, engaging in physical activity, establishing emergency distractions, utilizing visualization techniques, practicing progressive muscle relaxation, building a support system, developing positive affirmations, engaging in therapeutic techniques, setting and celebrating milestones, embracing self-compassion, and planning for difficult situations. The idea is to use a combination of these tactics that are particularly meaningful to you and connect with the specific characteristics of your recovery path.

Discuss the role of support systems, both professional and personal.

The importance of support systems in the complicated and difficult road of quitting porn addiction cannot be emphasized. Professional and personal support are critical in enabling individuals, particularly women, to traverse the path of recovery with resilience, understanding, and a fresh sense of hope.

Professional Assistance:

Therapeutic Direction:

Therapeutic advice is a cornerstone of professional support. Seeking the help of therapists, counselors, or addiction experts provides individuals with a secure and confidential environment in which to investigate the underlying issues that contribute to their addiction. Evidence-based modalities like as cognitive-behavioral therapy (CBT) or dialectical behavior therapy (DBT) are used by therapists to give individualized techniques for regulating triggers, resolving erroneous thought patterns, and creating healthy coping mechanisms.

Individualized Treatment Strategies:

Professional assistance facilitates the formulation of tailored treatment strategies. Recognizing that each person's path with addiction is unique, these programs target the individual's personal requirements, difficulties, and aspirations. The joint effort of the professional and the person seeking assistance results in the development of a roadmap that changes with the individual's success, generating a sense of ownership and empowerment.

Accountability and Progress Evaluation:

Professional support systems add accountability and progress tracking. Regular meetings with a therapist or counselor offer individuals with a structured framework in which to reflect on their experiences, track progress, and confront issues. This responsibility promotes persistent commitment to the recovery path and acts as a source of inspiration throughout both successes and disappointments.

Development of Skills and Coping Mechanisms:

Individuals are given vital skills and coping techniques by therapeutic specialists. These strategies help women manage triggers, negotiate desires, and deal with the emotional intricacies of addiction. Skill development becomes an important part of the rehabilitation process, empowering people with the resources they need to confront the difficulties ahead.

Personal Assistance

Friends and family:

Personal support systems, which include family and friends, lay the groundwork for understanding and empathy. Sharing one's experience with loved ones creates an environment in which people feel listened, appreciated, and supported. Family and friends become pillars of support, encouraging and motivating you through the ups and downs of the healing process.

Peer Support Organizations:

Peer support groups offer a distinct type of personal assistance. Connecting with others who are going through similar things fosters a sense of community and minimizes feelings of loneliness. Peer support groups provide a forum for sharing experiences, encouraging one another, and exchanging coping skills. This common journey strengthens the realization that individuals are not alone in their difficulties.

Validation on an emotional level:

Personal support systems provide emotional affirmation, which is essential in the rehabilitation process. Hearing and being understood by friends and family confirms the emotional intricacies of addiction. This emotional affirmation minimizes emotions of shame and guilt, fostering a healing and self-acceptance environment.

Practical Support:

Personal support networks can provide practical aid to alleviate the pressures of daily living. Whether it's assistance with duties, childcare, or providing a welcoming home atmosphere, practical support helps to reduce pressures that might aggravate addiction. This type of aid allows people to concentrate more completely on their recuperation.

Professional and Personal Support Working Together

Approach to Holistic Care:

The collaboration of professional and personal support networks enables a more comprehensive approach to care. Professionals give clinical competence and evidence-based therapies, whereas personal support networks provide empathy, unconditional love, and shared experiences. They work together to treat the many facets of addiction, fostering overall well-being.

Bridging Understanding Gaps:

Personal support networks frequently serve as understanding bridges between the person and the professional. Loved ones watch the day-to-day difficulties, offering crucial information that specialists may not notice during treatment sessions. By including the varied viewpoints of personal connections, this partnership improves the effectiveness of professional solutions.

Improving Accountability:

Accountability is improved by combining professional and personal assistance. Professionals provide organized advice, and personal support networks strengthen daily commitment to recovery. This dual accountability reinforces a person's determination while also providing a safety net that reduces the danger of relapse.

Creating an Empathy Culture:

A culture of empathy and understanding is fostered by the collaboration of professional and personal support networks. It promotes free communication by allowing people to discuss their worries, struggles, and triumphs without fear of being judged. This empathy culture fosters a supportive atmosphere in which individuals may tackle the complexity of addiction with courage and sincerity.

Finally, the complicated tapestry of overcoming porn addiction, as well as the interweaving strands of professional and personal support, provide a robust fabric on which individuals, particularly women, may rely. Collaboration among therapy experts, family, friends, and peer support groups tackles the many facets of addiction, encouraging a comprehensive and powerful approach to recovery.

Individuals may traverse the obstacles of addiction with strength, resilience, and a fresh sense of hope with professional supervision giving clinical knowledge and individualized therapies and personal support networks offering love, understanding, and daily encouragement. The collaboration of these support systems is an essential component of the transformational path toward long-term healing.

Chapter 5

Breaking the Cycle

We begin on the transforming process of ending the cycle of porn addiction in the critical chapter of this guide. This chapter acts as a compass, helping women through the complexities of breaking free from the bonds of addiction, cultivating resilience, self-empowerment, and pursuing a life of purpose and authenticity.

1. Recognizing the Patterns:

Recognizing the tendencies that have sustained the addiction is the first step in breaking the cycle. It entails a brave study of the recurrent behaviors, triggers, and emotional landscapes that keep the cycle going. This understanding serves as a catalyst for transformation, providing insights into the complex web of addiction.

Accepting Change as a Constant:

Breaking the loop necessitates a fundamental adjustment in viewpoint – accepting that change is not only essential, but also unavoidable. Accepting change as a constant encourages women to let go of old habits and explore the possibilities of transformation. Change becomes a traveling companion on the path to breaking free from the cycle of addiction.

Developing Resilience:

Breaking the pattern becomes dependent on resilience. This entails acquiring the ability to recover from failures, obstacles, and vulnerable times. Cultivating resilience equips women with the courage to confront the uncertainties of change, cultivating a mentality that sees problems as chances for growth rather than insurmountable hurdles.

Identity and Values Redefined:

Breaking out from the cycle of addiction necessitates a significant amount of self-discovery. It is necessary for women to reinvent their identities outside of the limits of addiction, embracing their innate value and potential. Clarifying personal values serves as a guiding light, assisting individuals in aligning their activities with a vision of a life full of meaning and authenticity.

Developing Healthy Habits:

Breaking the pattern requires incorporating good practices into daily living. Routines that promote physical well-being, mental health, and positive engagement lay the groundwork for long-term improvement. Healthy behaviors not only improve general well-being, but they also provide constructive alternatives to the addictive patterns.

Creating a Helpful Network:

Breaking the pattern requires a group effort. Creating and maintaining a supporting network that includes both professional and personal ties is crucial reinforcement. This network serves as a safety net, providing support, understanding, and accountability during times of vulnerability and triumph.

Face-to-Face with Triggers:

Breaking the loop requires confronting triggers straight on. This entails being proactive in recognizing and regulating triggers, applying coping methods, and handling difficult situations with resilience. Confrontation transforms into a transforming process that allows women to retake control over their reactions to triggers.

Celebrating Progress and Milestones:

Celebrating little victories is an important part of breaking the pattern. Recognizing and recognizing accomplishments along the way promotes a sense of accomplishment and inspiration. These commemorations function as liberation milestones, underlining the transforming power of devotion to change.

Learning from Mistakes:

Setbacks: Setbacks are an unavoidable aspect of the road to break the cycle. Instead of perceiving setbacks as failures, learning from them becomes a strong instrument for progress. Each setback serves as a lesson in resilience, self-awareness, and improving the tactics used to overcome obstacles.

Accepting Self-Compassion:

Breaking the pattern necessitates compassion for oneself. It is critical to embrace oneself with love throughout times of vulnerability, setbacks, or relapse. Self-compassion becomes a source of strength, guiding the internal dialogue toward optimism, comprehension, and dedication to the recovery process.

Personal Empowerment Reclaimed:

Breaking out from the cycle is an act of recovering personal power. It entails acknowledging that individuals have the power to mold their own destinies, make deliberate decisions, and live in accordance with their ideals. Reclaiming personal empowerment becomes the motivating factor behind the transforming journey toward long-term addiction freedom.

Outline a step-by-step plan for breaking the cycle of addiction.

Breaking the cycle of addiction is a transforming process that needs commitment, self-reflection, and deliberate action. This step-by-step method offers an organized roadmap for those, mainly women, who want to break free from the hold of porn addiction:

Recognize the Addiction:

Recognize and embrace the addiction's presence without judgment.

Recognize its influence on numerous elements of life, such as relationships, mental health, and general well-being.

Seek Professional Help:

Contact a therapist, counselor, or addiction specialist.

Collaborate with specialists to obtain insight into the fundamental causes of addiction.

Create a tailored treatment plan that fits your specific needs and goals.

Create a Support System:

Share your experience with trustworthy friends, family, and support groups.

Encourage open communication and the development of a supporting network that provides encouragement, understanding, and accountability.

Recognize Triggers and Patterns:

Conduct an in-depth self-evaluation to uncover addiction triggers and patterns.

Maintain a trigger notebook to record emotional states, events, and ideas before episodes of addictive behavior.

Create Coping Mechanisms:

Develop coping techniques customized to specific triggers in collaboration with specialists.

In order to regulate desires and negotiate difficult situations, use mindfulness practices, relaxation techniques, and healthy alternatives.

Define Your Boundaries:

Set clear and attainable limits for the intake of sexual content.

Communicate these limits to oneself as well as, if applicable, partners or close relationships.

Personal values must be redefined:

Engage in a self-discovery journey to clarify your values outside of the limits of addiction.

Clarify and prioritize values that are consistent with a vision of a life full of meaning and authenticity.

Establish a Structured Routine:

Create a daily regimen that reduces idle time and provides structure.

Incorporate good habits into the routine, such as frequent exercise, proper sleep, and pleasant hobbies.

Put in place technological safeguards:

To limit access to explicit content, use technology protections such as filters, parental controls, or accountability applications.

Make technology an ally in your recovery path.

Observe Milestones:

Set attainable goals and appreciate all achievements, no matter how minor.

Recognize and recognize accomplishments to promote a sense of success and drive.

Setbacks provide us valuable lessons:

Consider setbacks to be opportunities for learning and progress.

Analyze the events that led to setbacks and alter plans as needed.

Exercise Self-Compassion:

During difficult times, cultivate a self-compassionate perspective.

Kindly speak to oneself, realizing that the road includes both growth and failures.

Maintain Constant Self-Reflection:

Reflect on the trip on a regular basis, recognizing areas for improvement and areas that may require further focus.

Adjust the plan depending on changing requirements and self-reflection insights.

Reclaim Your Personal Power:

Recognize and reclaim your personal power as a change agent.

Accept the notion that individuals have the ability to mold their own destinies and make deliberate decisions.

Encourage a Life of Meaning and Authenticity:

Align your behaviors and decisions with your ideals.

Cultivate a life of meaning and honesty, strengthening your commitment to a life free of addiction.

This step-by-step method offers a complete roadmap for ending the addiction cycle. Individuals may traverse the intricacies of addiction with resilience, bravery, and a dedication to long-term recovery by combining professional help, a strong personal network, self-reflection, and deliberate activities

Discuss the importance of setting realistic goals and celebrating small victories.

The significance of establishing realistic objectives and appreciating minor accomplishments in the transforming process of addiction recovery cannot be emphasized. This dynamic pair is a strong motor moving individuals, particularly women struggling with porn addiction, toward long-term recovery. Understanding the relevance of these factors is critical for fostering resilience, drive, and a sense of success on the route to long-term transformation.

Setting Realistic Objectives:

Setting achievable goals is the foundation of a successful recovery journey. Goal-setting realism entails matching goals with the present stage of recovery, appreciating individual capacities, and realizing the multidimensional nature of addiction. Here's why setting realistic objectives is important:

Motivation and concentration:

Realistic objectives give a clear roadmap for motivation and attention. When people create attainable goals, the route forward becomes visible, generating a feeling of purpose and direction. This, in turn, increases devotion to the healing process.

Avoiding Overwhelm:

Overachieved ambitions can lead to overload, causing tension and worry. Realistic objectives, on the other hand, divide the rehabilitation process into achievable segments. This gradual approach reduces the possibility of feeling overwhelmed, allowing people to traverse the path with greater comfort.

Developing Self-Belief:

Achieving realistic goals helps to a consistent stream of accomplishments. Each accomplishment serves as a foundation for confidence, strengthening the conviction that change is possible. Confidence may be an effective antidote to the self-doubt that might precede addiction rehabilitation.

Keeping the Momentum:

Realistic goals keep momentum going by establishing a rhythm of development. Consistent forward action, even in little amounts, creates momentum that drives individuals through the hurdles of addiction recovery.

Small Victories to Celebrate:

Small triumphs are a powerful force that magnifies the impact of realistic goal-setting. These seemingly little triumphs serve as the foundation for resilience and motivation. Here are some of the reasons why celebrating little accomplishments is important during the healing process:

Using Positive Reinforcement:

Small triumphs provide real proof of progress. Recognizing and celebrating these accomplishments provides positive reinforcement, indicating to individuals that their efforts are having an impact. This positive feedback loop fortifies the determination to persevere in the face of adversity.

Developing a Positive Attitude:

Celebrating little accomplishments fosters a good attitude. Rather than concentrating on perceived inadequacies, this shift in viewpoint entails actively identifying and praising progress. A positive mentality becomes a driving force, creating the recovery journey's story.

Discouragement Reduction:

Addiction treatment is frequently laden with difficulties, and setbacks are unavoidable. Celebrating modest triumphs may be an effective way to counteract discouragement during challenging times. It provides a counterpoint to times of frustration by reminding people of their ability to succeed.

Developing Self-Compassion:

Small achievements provide people opportunity to cultivate self-compassion. Rather than harsh self-criticism, recognizing these accomplishments promotes a gentle and understanding internal conversation. Self-compassion is an essential component in developing resilience and emotional well-being.

Creating Progress Milestones:

Small triumphs add together to make progress milestones. These landmarks serve as defining markers on the path from addiction to recovery. Celebrating instills a sense of accomplishment, changing the healing process into a series of victories against adversity.

Finally, setting realistic objectives and recognizing little accomplishments are critical components of an addiction recovery path. Realistic objectives give a defined framework for motivation, overwhelm prevention, confidence development, and momentum maintenance. Celebrating little triumphs magnifies the effect of these goals by providing positive reinforcement, establishing a positive mentality, combating discouragement, encouraging self-compassion, and generating significant progress milestones. These factors work together to create a dynamic synergy that enables people to traverse the intricacies of addiction recovery with resilience, purpose, and a profound appreciation for the transformational potential of incremental achievement.

Emphasize the concept of progress, not perfection.

The motto "progress, not perfection" emerges as a guiding beacon in the multifaceted landscape of addiction recovery, particularly for women navigating the delicate obstacles of overcoming porn addiction. This notion represents a radical shift in viewpoint, stressing the transforming path of development, resilience, and self-discovery above the elusive chase of perfection.

Understanding Recovery's Imperfection:

The road to recovery from porn addiction is an inherently flawed one. With its complicated web of emotional, psychological, and sociological variables, addiction defies the idea of a linear and perfect road to recovery. Women facing this difficulty are frequently subjected to cultural standards and internalized pressures that demand perfection. Accepting the imperfections of rehabilitation becomes a critical step in removing these unreasonable expectations.

The Influence of Incremental Progress:

At the heart of "progress, not perfection" is the recognition that the recovery process is comprised of little steps. Setting reasonable and attainable goals becomes a pillar of growth. Whether it's cutting back on explicit content intake, getting professional help, or establishing healthier coping methods, each tiny step adds to the broader story of development.

The value of gradual progress rests in its capacity to inspire drive, minimize overwhelm, create confidence, and maintain momentum. Recognizing the value of incremental growth becomes a revolutionary act in a world preoccupied with instant satisfaction. It reframes the trip as a succession of attainable milestones, each one a testimonial to the individual's strength and dedication.

Navigating the Difficulties of Setbacks

Setbacks are not considered as failures in the quest of growth, but as necessary components of the healing process. Women facing porn addiction frequently confront periods of vulnerability and difficulty. In managing the intricacies of setbacks, progress, rather than perfection, becomes a guiding principle:

Possibilities for Learning:

Setbacks are considered as learning and growth opportunities rather than condemnations. Each setback reveals useful information about triggers, weaknesses, and areas that may require extra attention. Setbacks are transformed from barriers into stepping stones for long-term rehabilitation.

Resilience in the Face of Adversity:

Accepting progress rather than perfection fosters resilience. Women are urged to recover from failures, equipped with the knowledge that resilience is not the absence of obstacles, but the ability to adapt, learn, and persevere in the face of them. Resilience transforms into a source of empowerment and strength.

Perfectionist Stress Reduction:

On the road to recovery, perfectionism is a regular companion. The notion of progress, rather than perfection, relieves the demands that come with perfectionism. It enables women to let go of the demand for instant gratification and immaculate accomplishment, creating a more compassionate and realistic approach to their recovery path.

Embracing the Self-Discovery Process

Recovery is about reclaiming one's genuine self from the limits of addiction, not only abstaining from destructive activities. Progress, rather than perfection, becomes a guiding factor in this self-discovery process:

Identity Reconstruction:

Addiction is frequently connected with one's sense of self. Women are encouraged to reclaim their identities beyond the labels of addiction via progress, not perfection. It entails a thorough examination of one's personal beliefs, strengths, and objectives, enabling for the emergence of a more authentic self.

Cultivating Personal Development:

Personal development thrives on imperfection. Women managing the nuances of porn addiction face obstacles that require development. Instead of a destination, the notion of development, rather than perfection, depicts this evolution as an ongoing and dynamic process. It turns the emphasis away from perfection and toward human growth.

Stressing Resilience:

The imperfection of rehabilitation emphasizes the tenacity necessary to negotiate its twists and turns. Women are encouraged to appreciate their abilities to recover, adapt, and persevere in the face of adversity. Resilience becomes a badge of honor, demonstrating strength under adversity.

Creating a Community of Support

The idea of progress, rather than perfection, develops a sense of camaraderie among the recovery community. Women who are traveling together realize that perfection is an impossible goal. The emphasis on progress fosters mutual support, empathy, and appreciation of one another's accomplishments. The imperfections of the recovery process are acknowledged and cherished in this supportive group.

Finally, "progress, not perfection" emerges as a liberating ideology in the field of porn addiction rehabilitation for women. It frees women from the constraints of perfectionism, allowing them to embark on the flawed but transforming road of recovery. Women may promote resilience in the face of failures, foster personal growth, and create a supportive community that recognizes and celebrates the power found in imperfection by embracing progress. The phrase becomes a compass, directing women on a path of self-compassion, honesty, and the powerful realization that progress is a testimonial to strength, bravery, and the pursuit of a life beyond addiction.

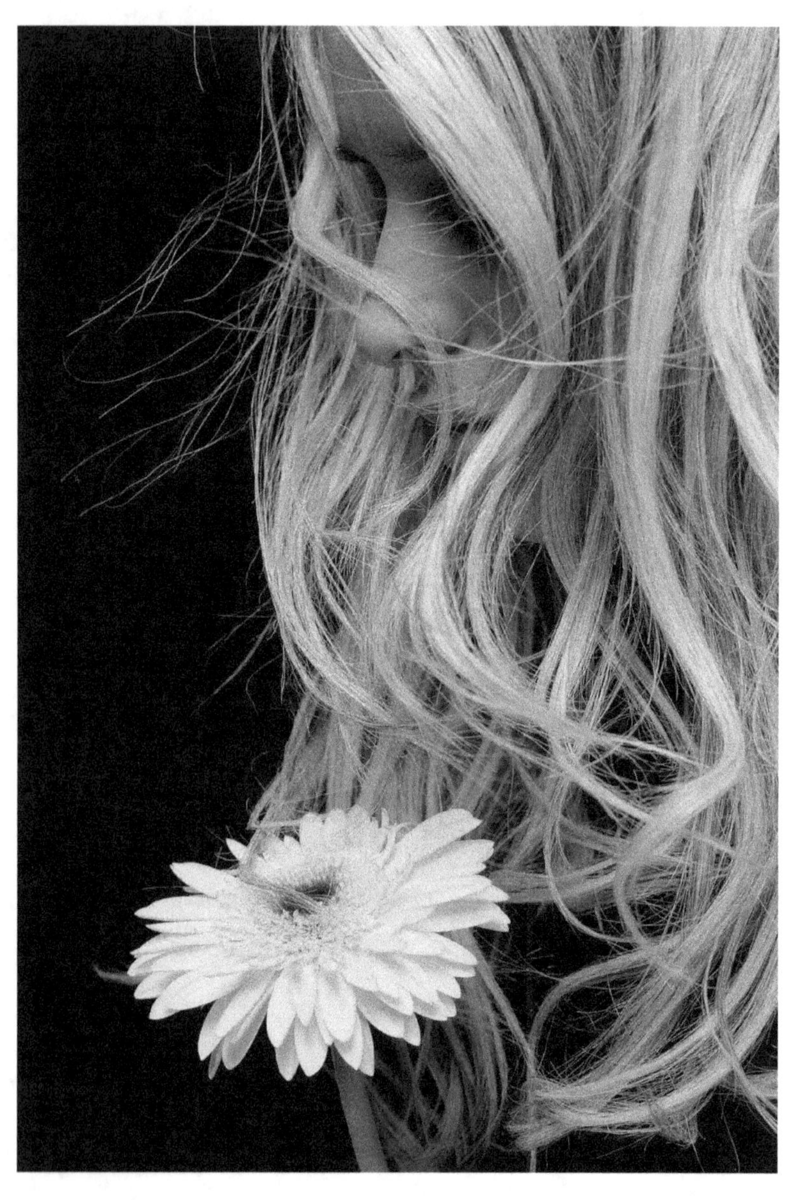

Chapter 6

Building a Healthy Relationship with Sexuality

We go into the critical topic of developing a healthy connection with sexuality in the final part of our transforming journey towards overcoming porn addiction. This chapter is intended to help women rediscover and rebuild their relationship with their own sexuality, establishing a positive and empowered narrative that transcends the shadows of addiction.

Accepting Sexual Wellness:

Building a healthy relationship with sexuality begins with a basic adjustment in perspective – understanding sexuality as an essential component of total health. Accept the notion that having a pleasant and meaningful sexual life is not only feasible, but also necessary for personal growth and well-being.

Self-Discovery and Self-Exploration:

Encourage women to go on a path of self-discovery and adventure. This requires them to reconnect with their own bodies, wants, and preferences. In recovering agency over one's sexuality, self-awareness becomes a valuable weapon.

Beyond Addiction, Redefining Sexuality:

Challenge the narratives and associations that may have developed during the addiction recovery process. Assist women in redefining their sexuality outside the constraints of prior experiences, realizing that they have the power to build a narrative that is consistent with their beliefs and objectives.

Communicating with Colleagues:

Building a successful sexual connection requires effective communication. Encourage couples to have open and honest talks about their wishes, boundaries, and shared expectations. Creating a secure environment for communication promotes mutual understanding and helps to maintain a pleasant sexual dynamic.

Intimacy Beyond the Screens:

One of the difficulties brought on by porn addiction is the possibility for alienation from real-life closeness. Women should be encouraged to discover intimacy outside screens and false portrayals. Genuine connection and emotional closeness are critical components of a good sexual relationship.

Mindfulness and Present Moment Awareness:

Introduce mindfulness practice into the arena of sexuality. Encourage being in the now and developing a stronger connection with feelings and emotions. Mindfulness enables women to have a deeper knowledge of their own wants and emotions.

Seeking Professional Help:

Recognize that developing a healthy sexual relationship may need obtaining professional help, such as therapy or counseling. Trained specialists can offer customized assistance in addressing individual difficulties and leading the process of sexual rediscovery.

Setting Healthy Boundaries:

Encourage women to set and discuss appropriate sexual limits. Recognize that setting limits is not only a right, but also an important part of developing a partnership that respects individual autonomy and comfort.

Sensuality Is Important:

Encourage sensuality to be celebrated as a pleasant and enriching component of life. Sensuality extends beyond the act of sex and includes appreciating the beauty of touch, connection, and the numerous ways in which people can feel pleasure.

Consent and respect are emphasized:

Consent and respect are non-negotiable when it comes to developing a healthy sexual relationship. In every element of a sexual relationship, emphasize the need of clear communication and mutual respect, producing an environment in which both lovers feel appreciated and understood.

Explore the idea of fostering a positive and healthy relationship with one's own sexuality.

Building a happy and healthy connection with one's own sexuality is a transformative and uplifting experience that extends beyond conquering obstacles. It entails self-reflection, self-acceptance, and deliberate efforts to rewrite the story of one's sexuality. Here are some important factors to consider while developing a happy and healthy relationship with your own sexuality.

Accept Self-Exploration:

Begin the journey by appreciating the beauty of self-discovery. Allow yourself time and space to become acquainted with your own body, wants, and boundaries. Self-exploration is a mental and emotional process that involves an honest and open communication with oneself.

Dispel Stigmas and Preconceptions:

Dispel cultural stigmas and misconceptions about sexuality. Recognize that sexuality is a normal and diverse part of the human experience. By challenging social standards and letting go of judgment, you create a more welcoming and positive environment for your own sexual identity.

Self-acceptance should be prioritized:

Embrace all aspects of your sexuality to practice self-acceptance. Recognize that your wants, tastes, and dreams are unique to you. Acceptance does not imply complying to external standards, but rather loving and accepting your real self.

Let Go of Guilt and Shame:

Addiction is frequently accompanied by feelings of guilt and shame. Release these negative feelings purposefully as you work to have a healthy relationship with your sexuality. Recognize that your past does not define you, and that by letting go of guilt and shame, you make room for development and healing.

Develop Your Mindfulness:

Incorporate awareness into your sexual encounters. Being totally present in the moment helps you to fully feel and appreciate the sensations, emotions, and relationships that are present. Mindfulness helps you have a better knowledge of your own wants and hastens your interaction with your sexuality.

Recognize the Influence of Media:

Recognize the impact of media, especially explicit material, on your sexuality perceptions. Recognize that the media frequently promotes unrealistic and sensationalized versions of sexual encounters. Recognizing this influence empowers you to build a more honest and positive image of your own sexuality.

Connect with Yourself:

Make open and honest conversation with oneself a habit. This entails becoming aware of your own feelings, wants, and boundaries. Actively listen to your own wants and preferences, building a self-awareness foundation that adds to a happy connection with your sexuality.

Sensuality should be celebrated:

Celebrate sensuality in all of its manifestations. Sensuality covers the beauty of touch, connection, and appreciation for one's own body in addition to the actual act of sex. By honoring sensuality, you move the emphasis away from performance and toward the overall experience of pleasure and connection.

Establish Limits:

Set firm and healthy boundaries for yourself. Recognize what feels comfortable and consensual in your sexual encounters. Setting limits is a powerful act that secures your well-being and helps you have a healthy and respectful connection with your sexuality.

Seek Professional Help:

Consider obtaining professional help to manage issues or explore parts of your sexuality if necessary. A qualified therapist or counselor may provide a secure, nonjudgmental environment for self-exploration, as well as help suited to your specific needs.

Provide guidance on rediscovering intimacy and connection.

Rediscovering intimacy and connection is a significant process that includes emotional, mental, and spiritual elements. Rebuilding personal ties may be transformational for people who have overcome the struggles of addiction. Here is a guide to help you through the process:

Develop Self-Compassion:

Begin with developing self-compassion. Recognize that the journey to regain intimacy is individualized, and that each person's route is distinguished by personal growth and healing. Accept yourself with kindness, knowing that self-compassion is the cornerstone for developing meaningful relationships with others.

Consider your personal values:

Consider your personal ideals and the qualities you desire in close relationships. Determine your own desires, limitations, and goals. Understanding your values creates the framework for genuine friendships that are consistent with your sense of self.

Create an Open Communication Environment:

The foundation of regaining intimacy is open communication. Make a secure environment for your spouse to have open and honest talks. Share your ideas, worries, and desires, allowing you to better understand each other's needs.

Accept Emotional Intimacy:

Recognize the value of emotional closeness. Emotional connection is the foundation of satisfying partnerships. Engage in activities that develop intimacy and understanding by encouraging vulnerability and emotional exchange.

Active listening should be practiced:

Improve your active listening skills. Show empathy and compassion by paying attention to your partner's ideas and feelings. By noticing and appreciating one other's opinions, active listening promotes a stronger relationship.

Combine Sensuality and Touch:

Discover sensuality and touch as intimate expressions. Engage in touch-related activities, such as holding hands, embracing, or simply being physically nearer. Sensual encounters help to foster a sense of connection and physical closeness.

Be in the Present Moment:

Accept awareness and live in the present moment. Focus on the present without concentrating on previous difficulties whether engaging in talks, sharing experiences, or being personal. Mindfulness improves the quality of relationships by encouraging a greater appreciation for shared experiences.

Investigate Common Interests:

Exploring similar hobbies and activities is part of rediscovering closeness. Find activities or interests that you both like and can participate in together. Shared experiences form relationships and enhance the link between spouses.

Seek Professional Help If Necessary:

If difficulties persist, consider obtaining expert assistance. A therapist or counselor may provide you advice that is targeted to your individual requirements and enable open conversation. Professional assistance can help you navigate the complications of regaining intimacy.

Encourage Mutual Trust:

Create and nurture mutual trust. Trust is the core of any intimate relationship, and reestablishing it after adversity takes time and persistence. To foster a sense of security and trust in the relationship, demonstrate dependability and honesty.

CONCLUSION

This approach to overcoming porn addiction for women is a transforming path that provides not only a stop of destructive habits but also empowerment through knowledge. Every chapter contributes to a comprehensive rehabilitation, from understanding addiction to practical control measures. It teaches women how to spot warning signals, deal with disappointments, and form healthy relationships, all while encouraging self-discovery. Beyond conquering addiction, the handbook redefines sexuality with positivity, honoring power and endurance. As the pages shut, the story echoes— a story of women reclaiming their lives, embracing honesty and connection. This book serves as a companion, encouraging women to liberty, self-love, and empowerment.

HAPPY FREE LIFE

www.ingramcontent.com/pod-product-compliance
Lightning Source LLC
Chambersburg PA
CBHW070901260726
48661CB00004B/1523